Worth & Wellness Journal

Amy Latta

DEDICATION

This book is dedicated to my LattaLuvs, whom I share my deepest thoughts and struggles, and yet you love me anyway. I have worked through much of this journal in my emails to all of you, and you have yet to run.

Thank you for bringing your love and honesty to the table every single day.

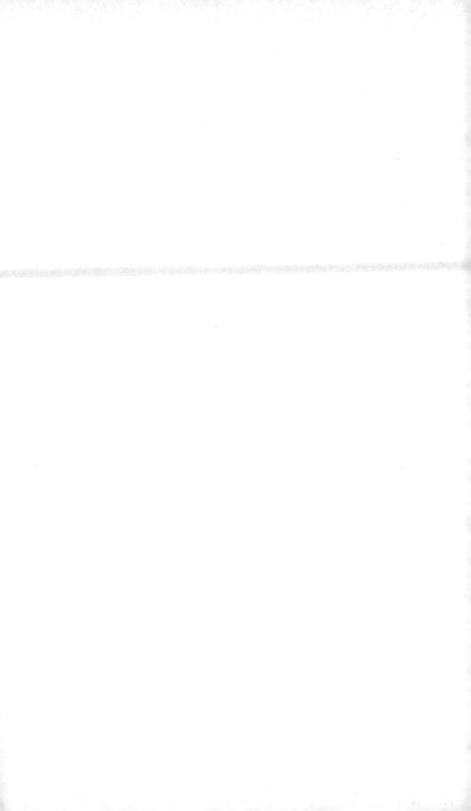

CONTENTS

ACKNOWLEDGMENTS

This journal would not have come together without the inspiration and help of the following:

1. My teachers, whose works I have read and studied; including Brooke Castillo, Brene Brown, Geneen Roth, Chalene Johnson, Dr. Wayne Dyer, Don Miguel Ruiz, Louise Hay, and Eckhart Tolle.

2. My mentor, Jennifer Mazella, for always providing a critical eye and helpful guidance.

3. My lobsters and closest confidants, Tammy Helfrich and Clay Shaver. You get me. Even when I do not.

4. Kelsey Humphreys and my Pursuit Mastermind. You make me want to be a better person.

5. Jon Acuff and the Dreamers & Builders. I wrote a book, guys. It is all your fault. Especially yours, Janeen. And you, too, Shayla.

6. One of my best friends, Melissa Boyer, whose one suggestion turned this from cumbersome tome to useful guide.

6. Extra special appreciation to my husband and children for putting up with me when I am in *creation mode.*

7. My mom. You are my biggest cheerleader of ever, and that is the best gift anyone has ever given me.

HOW TO USE THIS JOURNAL

Worth & Wellness Coaching utilizes the **Self-Fulfilling Prophecy Model**, which centers around this idea:
Circumstances are neutral, it is your thoughts about them that make them good or bad. These thoughts lead to feelings; feelings lead to actions; and actions give you your results, which often confirm your original thought.

Circumstances -> Thoughts -> Feelings -> Actions -> Results
This is the heart of why we do what we do.

This journal was created to help you become more aware of your thoughts and feelings on matters of health and fitness.

1. In the Wellness Focus, you will find daily nutrition, fitness, and self-care actions, plus space to add your own.

2. Modify the exercises to your fitness level by modifying the moves, breaking up reps throughout your day, or adding sets.

3. In the Worth Focus, tune into the thoughts and feelings that arise with each topic. Allow them to come to the surface, writing from a place of curiosity and non-judgment.

4. Use the Key Takeaways to highlight any surprises that arise, or to focus on the key thought that has held you back in the past.

5. Use the Mind-Mapping, Sketching, and Brainstorming Zone to draw or expand on any ideas that come to you.

Make your journal experience complete by visiting www.AmyLatta.com/30DayJournal to register to receive:

- Additional nutrition, fitness, and self-care action steps.
- Worth & Wellness goal tracker pack, including weekly goal sheets, meal planner, workout planner, and food lists.
- Access to the Worth & Wellness group on Facebook.

DAY ONE WELLNESS FOCUS

NUTRITION: Research five new recipes you would like to try.

___

FITNESS: 5 pushups, 20 crunches, 20 squats, :15s plank

___

SELF-CARE: Stand up taller and move with intention.

___

DAY ONE WORTH FOCUS

How does it feel to picture yourself taking on the goals you have set for this month?

___

___

___

___

___

___

___

___

___

___

___

___

What are your *Key Takeaways* to help you move forward?

_____

_____

_____

_____

_____

_____

_____

_____

MIND-MAPPING, SKETCHING, & BRAINSTORMING ZONE

DAY TWO WELLNESS FOCUS

NUTRITION: Make a weekly and monthly meal plan.

FITNESS: 10 jumping jacks, 10 mountain climbers, 5 burpees

SELF-CARE: Make sleep a priority. Allow for 7-9 hours each night.

DAY TWO WORTH FOCUS

Losing weight requires hard work and commitment. Are you ready to do things that are new or that you may not love?

_____

_____

_____

_____

_____

_____

_____

_____

_____

_____

_____

_____

_____

What are your *Key Takeaways* to help you move forward?

_____

_____

_____

_____

_____

_____

_____

_____

_____

MIND-MAPPING, SKETCHING, & BRAINSTORMING ZONE

DAY THREE WELLNESS FOCUS

NUTRITION: Remove the junk from your refrigerator and pantry.

FITNESS: 10 tricep dips, 20 bicycles, 20 lunges, :15s plank

SELF-CARE: Add 10 minutes of meditation or quiet time to the morning.

DAY THREE WORTH FOCUS

Curve balls are a part of life. How do you react when life does not go as planned?

_____

_____

_____

_____

_____

_____

_____

_____

_____

_____

_____

What are your *Key Takeaways* to help you move forward?

_____

_____

_____

_____

_____

_____

_____

_____

_____

MIND-MAPPING, SKETCHING, & BRAINSTORMING ZONE

DAY FOUR WELLNESS FOCUS
NUTRITION: Restock! Go shop for ingredients to the new recipes.

FITNESS: (Rest)

SELF-CARE: Make a list of positive things about yourself that have nothing to do with your body.

DAY FOUR WORTH FOCUS
What does your life look like in a perfect world? How do you feel about setting big audacious goals for yourself?

What are your *Key Takeaways* to help you move forward?

_____

_____

_____

_____

_____

_____

_____

_____

MIND-MAPPING, SKETCHING, & BRAINSTORMING ZONE

DAY FIVE WELLNESS FOCUS

NUTRITION: Drink half your body weight in ounces of water. (150lbs=75oz)

FITNESS: 7 pushups, 30 crunches, 30 squats, :30s plank

SELF-CARE: Take an hour-long "no electronics" break.

DAY FIVE WORTH FOCUS

Which scares you more - making big changes in your life or staying exactly where you are?

What are your *Key Takeaways* to help you move forward?

_____

_____

_____

_____

_____

_____

_____

_____

MIND-MAPPING, SKETCHING, & BRAINSTORMING ZONE

DAY SIX WELLNESS FOCUS
NUTRITION: Calculate your daily protein requirements.

FITNESS: 12 jumping jacks, 12 mountain climbers, 7 burpees

SELF-CARE: Get up and move at least 5 minutes every hour.

DAY SIX WORTH FOCUS
We are not guaranteed time on this Earth. How would you assess your life if today was your last day here? What would you change?

What are your *Key Takeaways* to help you move forward?

_____

_____

_____

_____

_____

_____

_____

_____

_____

MIND-MAPPING, SKETCHING, & BRAINSTORMING ZONE

DAY SEVEN WELLNESS FOCUS
NUTRITION: Add protein to your breakfast this morning.

FITNESS: 12 tricep dips, 25 bicycles, 25 lunges, :30s plank

SELF-CARE: Get out in nature! Take a 15 minute walk.

DAY SEVEN WORTH FOCUS
Healthy and fit looks different on everyone. How does it look on you?

What are your *Key Takeaways* to help you move forward?

_____

_____

_____

_____

_____

_____

_____

_____

_____

MIND-MAPPING, SKETCHING, & BRAINSTORMING ZONE

DAY EIGHT WELLNESS FOCUS

NUTRITION: Add berries to your breakfast and/or lunch.

FITNESS: (Rest)

SELF-CARE: Add 10 minutes of stretching to your morning.

DAY EIGHT WORTH FOCUS

Losing weight does not fix the problems of our life. What expectations are you putting on your weight loss?

What are your *Key Takeaways* to help you move forward?

_____

_____

_____

_____

_____

_____

_____

_____

MIND-MAPPING, SKETCHING, & BRAINSTORMING ZONE

DAY NINE WELLNESS FOCUS

NUTRITION: Try a completely new-to-you food.

_____

FITNESS: 10 pushups, 40 crunches, 40 squats, :45s plank

_____

SELF-CARE: Spend a few extra moments getting ready and put your best foot forward today.

_____

DAY NINE WORTH FOCUS

You are made for greater things than obsessing over the scale and calories. How does letting go of number tracking feel?

_____

_____

_____

_____

_____

_____

_____

_____

_____

_____

What are your *Key Takeaways* to help you move forward?

_____

_____

_____

_____

_____

_____

_____

_____

MIND-MAPPING, SKETCHING, & BRAINSTORMING ZONE

DAY TEN WELLNESS FOCUS
NUTRITION: Cut out all added and refined sugars.

FITNESS: 20 minute HiiT workout

SELF-CARE: Get creative - write, draw, design, compose, or color.

DAY TEN WORTH FOCUS
Perfection cannot be maintained. Where do you fall on the pendulum between perfection and not caring at all?

What are your *Key Takeaways* to help you move forward?

_____

_____

_____

_____

_____

_____

_____

_____

MIND-MAPPING, SKETCHING, & BRAINSTORMING ZONE

DAY ELEVEN WELLNESS FOCUS
NUTRITION: Drink 8-16oz of water upon waking.

FITNESS: 15 tricep dips, 30 bicycles, 30 lunges, :45s plank

SELF-CARE: Make your bedroom your sanctuary.

DAY ELEVEN WORTH FOCUS
What you have done in the past is not as important as what you do moving forward. Can you show yourself grace for past mistakes?

_____

_____

_____

_____

_____

_____

_____

_____

_____

_____

_____

_____

What are your *Key Takeaways* to help you move forward?

_____

_____

_____

_____

_____

_____

_____

_____

MIND-MAPPING, SKETCHING, & BRAINSTORMING ZONE

DAY TWELVE WELLNESS FOCUS

NUTRITION: Mix it up! Try an out-of-the-ordinary salad today.

FITNESS: (Rest)

SELF-CARE: Spend time doing something you love.

DAY TWELVE WORTH FOCUS

Sometimes foods we love make our bodies feel physically bad. How does not eating them feel?

_____

_____

_____

_____

_____

_____

_____

_____

_____

_____

_____

_____

What are your *Key Takeaways* to help you move forward?

_____

_____

_____

_____

_____

_____

_____

_____

_____

MIND-MAPPING, SKETCHING, & BRAINSTORMING ZONE

DAY THIRTEEN WELLNESS FOCUS
NUTRITION: Swap butter or oil for coconut oil in your cooking.

FITNESS: 12 pushups, 50 crunches, 50 squats, :60s plank

SELF-CARE: Notice any negative self-talk, and turn it positive.

DAY THIRTEEN WORTH FOCUS
We know most everything we need to get healthy and fit. What has kept you from implementing that knowledge?

What are your *Key Takeaways* to help you move forward?

_____

_____

_____

_____

_____

_____

_____

_____

MIND-MAPPING, SKETCHING, & BRAINSTORMING ZONE

DAY FOURTEEN WELLNESS FOCUS
NUTRITION: Add greens to each meal.

FITNESS: 15 jumping jacks, 15 mountain climbers, 10 burpees

SELF-CARE: Connect with someone in-real-life.

DAY FOURTEEN WORTH FOCUS
The world needs you, not some cheap imitation of someone else. How does it feel to just "do you?"

What are your *Key Takeaways* to help you move forward?

_____

_____

_____

_____

_____

_____

_____

_____

MIND-MAPPING, SKETCHING, & BRAINSTORMING ZONE

DAY FIFTEEN WELLNESS FOCUS

NUTRITION: Skip restaurants and take-out, and cook your own meals.

_____

FITNESS: 17 tricep dips, 35 bicycles, 35 lunges, :60s plank

_____

SELF-CARE: Try a fun new Thing to Do

_____

DAY FIFTEEN WORTH FOCUS

You cannot control how other people interpret you. How does it feel to know that someone does not like you?

_____

_____

_____

_____

_____

_____

_____

_____

_____

_____

_____

What are your *Key Takeaways* to help you move forward?

_____

_____

_____

_____

_____

_____

_____

_____

MIND-MAPPING, SKETCHING, & BRAINSTORMING ZONE

DAY SIXTEEN WELLNESS FOCUS
NUTRITION: Swap salt for a variety of herbs.

FITNESS: (Rest)

SELF-CARE: Write down five things to be happy about right now.

DAY SIXTEEN WORTH FOCUS
Exercise is a gift we give our bodies. What reasons do you have for not moving your body every day?

What are your *Key Takeaways* to help you move forward?

_____

_____

_____

_____

_____

_____

_____

_____

_____

MIND-MAPPING, SKETCHING, & BRAINSTORMING ZONE

DAY SEVENTEEN WELLNESS FOCUS
NUTRITION: Learn about eating for your hormone health.

FITNESS: 15 pushups, 60 crunches, 60 squats, :75s plank

SELF-CARE: Clear clutter by donating a box of things you no longer use.

DAY SEVENTEEN WORTH FOCUS
We have all been gifted with something that we are meant to share with the world. What is your gift and how do you share it?

What are your *Key Takeaways* to help you move forward?

_____

_____

_____

_____

_____

_____

_____

_____

_____

MIND-MAPPING, SKETCHING, & BRAINSTORMING ZONE

DAY EIGHTEEN WELLNESS FOCUS

NUTRITION: Add magnesium-rich foods to your diet.

FITNESS: 17 jumping jacks, 17 mountain climbers, 12 burpees

SELF-CARE: Perform a random act of kindness for someone.

DAY EIGHTEEN WORTH FOCUS

You are born with innate worth. It is there even if you cannot see it. Do you see your own worth?

What are your *Key Takeaways* to help you move forward?

_____

_____

_____

_____

_____

_____

_____

_____

MIND-MAPPING, SKETCHING, & BRAINSTORMING ZONE

DAY NINETEEN WELLNESS FOCUS
NUTRITION: Eat something you absolutely love today.

FITNESS: 20 tricep dips, 40 bicycles, 40 lunges, :75s plank

SELF-CARE: Give yourself a spa day at home.

DAY NINETEEN WORTH FOCUS
Failure is not avoidable, it is inevitable. I give you permission to fail. How does failure feel to you?

What are your *Key Takeaways* to help you move forward?

_____

_____

_____

_____

_____

_____

_____

_____

MIND-MAPPING, SKETCHING, & BRAINSTORMING ZONE

DAY TWENTY WELLNESS FOCUS

NUTRITION: Get more energy by eating your B-vitamins.

FITNESS: (Rest)

SELF-CARE: Bring positive energy into every room you enter.

DAY TWENTY WORTH FOCUS

There is power in "Me, too!" What can community allow you to do that you would not do otherwise?

What are your *Key Takeaways* to help you move forward?

_____

_____

_____

_____

_____

_____

_____

_____

MIND-MAPPING, SKETCHING, & BRAINSTORMING ZONE

DAY TWENTY-ONE WELLNESS FOCUS
NUTRITION: Eat more plant-based foods.

_____

FITNESS: 17 pushups, 70 crunches, 70 squats, :90s plank

_____

SELF-CARE: Spend 10mins in meditation or quiet time before bed.

_____

DAY TWENTY-ONE WORTH FOCUS
If you fail to plan, you are planning to fail. What prevents you from making a basic weekly eating and workout plan?

_____

_____

_____

_____

_____

_____

_____

_____

_____

_____

_____

What are your *Key Takeaways* to help you move forward?

_____

_____

_____

_____

_____

_____

_____

_____

MIND-MAPPING, SKETCHING, & BRAINSTORMING ZONE

DAY TWENTY-TWO WELLNESS FOCUS

NUTRITION: Spice it up with metabolism-boosting foods.

FITNESS: 20 minute HiiT workout

SELF-CARE: Write a list of boundaries for people in your life that violate your space. Communicate them.

DAY TWENTY-TWO WORTH FOCUS

Routines help make the daily tasks of getting and staying healthy significantly easier. How are you at daily wellness routines?

_____

_____

_____

_____

_____

_____

_____

_____

_____

_____

_____

_____

_____

What are your *Key Takeaways* to help you move forward?

_____

_____

_____

_____

_____

_____

_____

_____

MIND-MAPPING, SKETCHING, & BRAINSTORMING ZONE

DAY TWENTY-THREE WELLNESS FOCUS
NUTRITION: Remove all packaged foods today.

FITNESS: 22 tricep dips, 45 bicycles, 45 lunges, :90s plank

SELF-CARE: Get outside and spend time in nature.

DAY TWENTY-THREE WORTH FOCUS
Emotional eating is one of the biggest factors in weight struggles. What types of emotions do you eat from?

What are your *Key Takeaways* to help you move forward?

_____

_____

_____

_____

_____

_____

_____

_____

_____

MIND-MAPPING, SKETCHING, & BRAINSTORMING ZONE

DAY TWENTY-FOUR WELLNESS FOCUS
NUTRITION: Add good bacteria, such as Greek yogurt and probiotics

---

FITNESS: (Rest)

SELF-CARE: Slow down today and tune into your surroundings.

DAY TWENTY-FOUR WORTH FOCUS
Our happiness cannot depend on the actions of others. How much power do you give to other people in how you feel?

What are your *Key Takeaways* to help you move forward?

_____

_____

_____

_____

_____

_____

_____

_____

_____

MIND-MAPPING, SKETCHING, & BRAINSTORMING ZONE

DAY TWENTY-FIVE WELLNESS FOCUS
NUTRITION: Try high-protein grains, such as quinoa.

FITNESS: 20 pushups, 80 crunches, 80 squats, :120s plank

SELF-CARE: Watch your favorite movie.

DAY TWENTY-FIVE WORTH FOCUS
Sometimes we need to pull back so that we can spring forward. How comfortable are you to allow yourself rest?

_____

_____

_____

_____

_____

_____

_____

_____

_____

_____

_____

_____

_____

_____

What are your *Key Takeaways* to help you move forward?

_____

_____

_____

_____

_____

_____

_____

_____

MIND-MAPPING, SKETCHING, & BRAINSTORMING ZONE

DAY TWENTY-SIX WELLNESS FOCUS
NUTRITION: Remove diet and reduced-fat foods.

FITNESS: 20 jumping jacks, 20 mountain climbers, 15 burpees

SELF-CARE: Write a Thank You note to your biggest cheerleader.

DAY TWENTY-SIX WORTH FOCUS
Feelings do not define you, the type of person you are, or your worth. Are you afraid of your feelings or do you embrace them?

_____

_____

_____

_____

_____

_____

_____

_____

_____

_____

_____

_____

What are your *Key Takeaways* to help you move forward?

_____

_____

_____

_____

_____

_____

_____

_____

_____

MIND-MAPPING, SKETCHING, & BRAINSTORMING ZONE

DAY TWENTY-SEVEN WELLNESS FOCUS
NUTRITION: Create a list of healthy go-to meals to have on hand.

FITNESS: 25 tricep dips, 50 bicycles, 50 lunges, :120s plank

SELF-CARE: Smile at everyone you see.

DAY TEWNTY-SEVEN WORTH FOCUS
Comparison is the thief of joy, and either makes you feel superior or inferior. What comparisons do you make with others?

What are your *Key Takeaways* to help you move forward?

_____

_____

_____

_____

_____

_____

_____

_____

_____

MIND-MAPPING, SKETCHING, & BRAINSTORMING ZONE

DAY TWENTY-EIGHT WELLNESS FOCUS
NUTRITION: Revamp your favorite meal with healthier substitutions.

FITNESS: (Rest)

SELF-CARE: Sing and dance to your favorite song or playlist.

DAY TWENTY-EIGHT WORTH FOCUS
We often insist that others see things the way we see them. How do you let other people's opinions affect you?

What are your *Key Takeaways* to help you move forward?

_____

_____

_____

_____

_____

_____

_____

_____

_____

MIND-MAPPING, SKETCHING, & BRAINSTORMING ZONE

DAY TWENTY-NINE WELLNESS FOCUS

NUTRITION: Try green or white tea instead of coffee or soda.

FITNESS: 25 pushups, 90 crunches, 90 squats, :180s plank

SELF-CARE: Watch a funny movie and laugh until you cry.

DAY TWENTY-NINE WORTH FOCUS

We all have access to the same number of hours in a day. How do you feel about how you utilize your day?

What are your *Key Takeaways* to help you move forward?

_____

_____

_____

_____

_____

_____

_____

_____

MIND-MAPPING, SKETCHING, & BRAINSTORMING ZONE

DAY THIRTY WELLNESS FOCUS

NUTRITION: Add lemon water to your before-breakfast routine.

FITNESS: 25 jumping jacks, 25 mountain climbers, 20 burpees

SELF-CARE: Practice gratitude by making a list of 10 things you want in your life, that you already have.

DAY THIRTY WORTH FOCUS

Every endeavor can be a good experience, even if you are not successful. What can you learn from your failed attempts?

What are your *Key Takeaways* to help you move forward?

_____

_____

_____

_____

_____

_____

_____

_____

MIND-MAPPING, SKETCHING, & BRAINSTORMING ZONE

ABOUT THE AUTHOR

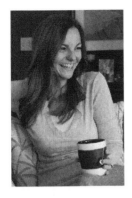 I have hated my thighs since sixth grade; and spent most of my 41 years unsure of who I was, a people pleaser paralyzed by fear.

Thanks to the works of the teachers I mention in the Acknowledgements, I learned to love my body as it was made, to stand tall in my authenticity, and embracing my Brave, my Silly, and my Worthy.

I write, coach, and speak to women exhausted by years of endless dieting, teaching them to change their bodies by first changing their mindset.

I am a total nerd who loves Star Wars, Sherlock, Supernatural, and The Walking Dead, and has a Dave Matthews Band fire dancer sticker on the family grocery-getter. I have a red lotus flower tattooed on my wrist, and love gerbera daisies, guacamole, and anything teal.

The folks that have to put up with my awkward realness include my ridiculously amazing husband, my lovely stepdaughter, and my two rambunctious yet thoughtful young boys. We live in Missouri, along with The Chubby Chihuahua, aka Lou.

This life ain't always pretty. But it is mine, and that is all that matters.

xoxo,

Amy

www.AmyLatta.com

Made in the USA
San Bernardino, CA
08 January 2016